Keto Breakfast

Ketogenic Diet Breakfast Recipes

Your Free Gifts

As a way of thanking you for the purchase, I'd like to offer you 2 complimentary gifts:

- **How To Get Through Any Weight Loss Plateau While On The Ketogenic Diet:** The title is self-explanatory; if you are struggling with getting off a weight loss plateau while on the Keto diet, you will find this free gift very eye opening on what has been ailing you. Grab your copy now by clicking/tapping here or simply enter http://bit.ly/2fantonpubketo into your browser.

- **5 Pillar Life Transformation Checklist:** This short book is about life transformation, presented in bit size pieces for easy implementation. I believe that without such a checklist, you are likely to have a hard time implementing anything in this book and any other thing you set out to do religiously and sticking to it for the long haul. It doesn't matter whether your goals relate to weight loss, relationships, personal finance, investing, personal development, improving communication in your family, your overall health, finances, improving your sex life, resolving issues in your relationship, fighting PMS successfully, investing, running a successful business, traveling etc. With a checklist like this one, you can bet that anything you do will seem a lot easier to implement until the end. Therefore, even if you don't continue reading this book, at least read the one thing that will help you in every other aspect of your life. Grab your copy now by clicking/tapping here or simply enter http://bit.ly/2fantonfreebie into your browser. Your life will never be the same again (if you implement what's in this book), I promise.

PS: I'd like your feedback. If you are happy with this book, please leave a review on Amazon.

Introduction

There is a reason they say breakfast is the most important meal of the day, which is why they also say we should eat breakfast like Kings. Nutritionists and different scientific studies always recommend that we all eat our breakfast. That is backed by statistics that have concluded that people who eat breakfast are significantly thinner than those who skip it.

The explanation to that is that given that you've gone without food for a number of hours while you were asleep, this means that your body is primed for optimal metabolic performance so what you eat will be used optimally.

The question that may be going through your mind is; **which foods are you going to eat for breakfast if you are on a Ketogenic diet**, *which prohibits eating wheat and grains as well as their products like bread, pancakes etc. as well as many other foods like cereals, which are rich in carbohydrates?*

Well, if you are having a hard time finding a variety of breakfast recipes while you are on a Ketogenic diet, this book is here for you.

The book aims to provide you with delicious and healthy Ketogenic breakfast recipes complete with nutritional information and total cook time. The recipes are categorized based on food types and method of preparation to help you easily try them!

More precisely, this book will show you:

- Omelets, frittatas and various egg dishes you can prepare while on the keto diet

- **Breakfast casseroles that you can prepare while on the keto diet**

- Breakfast recipes you can prepare using an instant pot while on the keto diet

- **Breakfast salads and side dishes that you can prepare on the keto diet**

- Delicious breads and pastries you can make while on the keto diet

- **Burgers, sandwiches and different breakfast meats you can prepare while on the keto diet**

- Pancakes and waffles that you can prepare while on the Ketogenic diet

- **And much, much more!**

After reading this book, you will have no reason why you should be eating the same old breakfast recipes when this book provides over 60 recipes to get you started!

Let's get started!

Keto Diet Breakfast Recipes

Copyright 2018 by Fantonpublishers.com - All rights reserved.

Table of Contents

Your Free Gifts ---------------------------------- **2**

Introduction ------------------------------------- **4**

Omelets, Frittatas and Egg Dishes ------------ **13**

   Bacon Spinach Egg Cup-------------------------------- *13*

   Italian Baked Eggs in Marinara Sauce ---------- *16*

   Spinach and Mozzarella Frittata ---------- *20*

   Shakshouka Skillet -----------------------------*22*

   Spicy Veggie Omelet --------------------------------*24*

   Chive and Cream Cheese Omelet------------------*25*

   Cheesy Italian Omelet ------------------------------ *27*

   Baked Eggs in Portobello Mushroom Caps------*29*

   Baked Star Squash & Eggs-------------------- *31*

   Heirloom Tomato and Swiss chard Eggs Benedict --*32*

Breakfast Casseroles ----------------------------**35**

   Savory Breakfast Casserole ----------------------*35*

   Yellow Squash Casserole---------------------------*37*

   Crock Pot Mexican Breakfast Casserole ---------*39*

   Crockpot Breakfast Casserole -------------------- *41*

   Sausage and Asparagus Casserole ---------------*43*

   Easy Breakfast Casserole --------------------------*45*

Breakfast Mock Casserole -------------------- *47*
Egg Casserole with Sausage and Cheese -------- *49*
Overnight Breakfast Casserole ------------------- *52*

Instant Pot Recipes --------------------------------- **54**
Breakfast Sandwich -------------------------------- *54*
Egg Muffins in the Pressure Cooker ------------- *56*
Keto Friendly Cornish Hens ---------------------- *58*
Eggs en Cocotte in the Instant Pot --------------- *60*
Crust-less Meat Lovers Quiche ------------------- *62*
Pressure Cooker Banana Bread ------------------ *64*
Instant Pot Mug Cakes ---------------------------- *67*
Korean Style Steamed Eggs ---------------------- *69*

Breakfast Salads & Side Dishes ----------------- **71**
Breakfast Spinach Salad --------------------------- *71*
Warming Breakfast Salad ------------------------- *73*
Canadian Bacon & Asparagus Salad ------------- *75*
Lemon Garlic Mushrooms salad ------------------ *77*
Greek Salad -- *79*
Greek Beef Salad ----------------------------------- *81*
Artichoke, Edamame, and Asparagus Salad --- *83*
A Skinny Caesar ------------------------------------ *85*
Blackened Chicken Salad with Tomato Chutney *88*

Breads and Pastries --------------------------- **90**

Crockpot Breakfast Meatloaf---------------------- 90

Keto Mini Meatloaves ------------------------------92

Grain-free Blueberry Muffin ----------------------94

Keto Lemon Poppy-seed Muffins ------------------96

Bacon cheeseburger Quiche -----------------------98

Keto Salmon & Cream Cheese Mug Muffin ---- 100

Low carb Taco Egg Muffins --------------------- 102

Shell Cheese Taco Cups--------------------------- 104

Avocado & Bacon Muffins ----------------------- 106

Burgers, Sandwiches and Breakfast Meats -- 108

Turkey Crusted Crockpot Breakfast ------------ 108

Bacon Bread Sandwich ---------------------------110

Keto Breakfast Burger---------------------------112

Keto Sausage Breakfast Sandwich --------------114

Breakfast Meat Bagel ------------------------------116

Chicken and Apple Sausage ----------------------118

Turkey Low Carb Sausage ---------------------- 120

Pancakes and Waffles ---------------------------121

Fluffy Keto Waffle ---------------------------------121

Flour-Less Pancakes------------------------------ 123

Pancakes with Blueberries ----------------------- 124

Kitchen Pumpkin Waffles------------------- 126

Pecan Hotcakes with Mixed Berries ----- *128*

Blueberries & Cream Crepes ---------------------- *130*

Eggs Benedict Zucchini Pancakes --------------- *132*

Conclusion -- **135**

Do You Like My Book & Approach To Publishing? ---------------------------------------**136**

1: First, I'd Love It If You Leave a Review of This Book on Amazon. ---------------------------------- *136*

2: Check Out My Other Keto Diet Books ------- *136*

3: Let's Get In Touch ------------------------------ *138*

4: Grab Some Freebies On Your Way Out; Giving Is Receiving, Right? ------------------------------ *138*

5: Suggest Topics That You'd Love Me To Cover To Increase Your Knowledge Bank. ------------- *139*

PSS: Let Me Also Help You Save Some Money! ---**140**

PS:

I have special interest in the Ketogenic diet. My wife has been following the Ketogenic diet and I can honestly say that the journey has been amazing. The diet works. And this is why I have committed to writing and publishing as many of the Ketogenic diet books as possible to give readers different options as far as the Ketogenic diet is concerned.

For instance, I have Ketogenic diet books exclusively dedicated for:

- Breakfast
- Main Meals
- Snacks
- Desserts
- Appetizers
- Soups
- Vegetarians
- Crockpot/slow cooker users
- Instant pot users
- Air fryer users
- People who are on the Paleo diet
- People who are following intermittent fasting

- People who are following carb cycling

And much more.

You can check out my [Ketogenic Diet Books fan page shop](#) for more of the books, as I continue publishing more and more. If you want me to add your category of the Ketogenic diet books that I have published so far, make sure to send me a message. I will do the heavy lifting for you and get back to you with a book that you will love.

You could also subscribe to my newsletter to receive updates whenever I have something new: http://bit.ly/2Cketodietfanton.

Omelets, Frittatas and Egg Dishes

Bacon Spinach Egg Cup

Prep Time: 15 minutes

Cook Time: 40 minutes

Total Time: 55 minutes

Serves 6

Directions

6 eggs

2 slices onions, chopped

4 mushrooms, chopped

1 1/4 cups shredded Colby-jack cheese, divided

1 pinch salt and ground black pepper

1 pinch onion powder

1/2 (12-ounce) package frozen chopped spinach

1 tablespoon heavy whipping cream

4 slices thick-cut bacon, diced

1/4 green bell pepper, chopped

1/2 teaspoon salt

1/4 teaspoon ground black pepper

1 pinch garlic powder

Directions

1. Preheat your oven to 350ºF and then coat 12 muffin cups using some cooking spray.

2. Over medium-high heat, cook the bacon in a skillet until crisp for around 10 minutes, while stirring.

3. Once set, put the bacon in a separate bowl but reserve the bacon grease in the skillet.

4. In the skillet that has reserved grease, combine onion, green bell pepper, salt, spinach, ground pepper and mushrooms.

5. Cook the mixture for about 5 minutes to soften then transfer this mixture into a separate bowl. Refrigerate for around 5 minutes.

6. In a bowl, whisk together cream and eggs and then stir 1 cup Jack cheese, onion powder, ¼-teaspoon ground pepper, garlic powder and ½ teaspoon salt.

7. Remove the veggies from the freezer and add to the egg mixture alongside the bacon. Mix gently to incorporate.

8. At this point, scoop ¼ cup of the egg mixture into each muffin cup, and then top each using the remaining cheese.

9. Finally bake for around 20 minutes or until the egg cups are just set.

Keto Diet Breakfast Recipes

Calories 237, Carbs 4g, Protein 16.5g, Fat 17.7g

Italian Baked Eggs in Marinara Sauce

Prep Time: 10 minutes

Cook Time: 12 minutes

Total Time: 22 minutes

Serves 1

Ingredients

2 tablespoons heavy whipping cream

1/3 cup of homemade marinara sauce (recipe below)

1 tablespoons finely shredded cheese

½ teaspoon red pepper flakes

Salt

Freshly ground black pepper

1 ½ teaspoons chopped fresh flat-leaf parsley

2 eggs

2 teaspoons olive oil

Directions

1. Preheat your oven to 400º F.

2. Then spoon the marinara sauce in a baking dish, to about ¼ inch high from the bottom. Sprinkle with parsley, red pepper flakes, black pepper and salt.

3. At the center of the sauce, make a narrow well to hold the eggs. Once done, crack in the eggs into a ramekin and then pour over the sauce.

4. Sprinkle with the cheese, cream and olive oil and season with pepper and salt.

5. At this point, bake in the preheated oven until the egg yolks are set or for around 10 to 12 minutes.

Calories 549, Carbs 9.5g, Protein 24.4g, Fat 37.3g

Keto Friendly Marinara Sauce

Prep Time: 5 minutes

Cook Time: 0 minutes

Total Time: 5 minutes

Yields: 4 cups

Ingredients

1 teaspoon of dried parsley

1 teaspoon of dried oregano

1 teaspoon of dried basil

1 teaspoon of garlic powder

1 teaspoon of onion powder

½ teaspoon red pepper flakes

¼ teaspoon of black pepper

¼ cup of extra virgin olive oil

1 tablespoon of red wine vinegar

28 ounce can of peeled organic tomatoes with no sugar added (you can use normal tomatoes)

Salt to taste

Directions

Simply puree olive oil, tomatoes along with any liquids from the can into a blender then stir in the other ingredients and continue blending until everything is nicely mixed. Taste for seasoning and adjust if necessary.

Calories per ½ cup serving: Calories 84, Protein 1g, Carb 3g net, Fat 7

Note: You will need this recipe multiple times when making different ingredients that call for tomato or marinara sauce in the book so when I mention tomato sauce or marinara sauce anywhere else in the book, refer to this recipe.

Spinach and Mozzarella Frittata

Prep Time: 15 minutes

Cook Time: 90 minutes

Total Time: 1 hour 15 minutes

Serves 3

Ingredients

2 Roma tomatoes, diced

Salt to taste

2 cups chopped baby spinach, without stems

½ teaspoon white pepper

1/2 teaspoon black pepper

4 tablespoons 1% milk

3 egg whites

6 eggs

2 cups 2% shredded mozzarella cheese, divided

1 cup diced onion

2 tablespoons extra-virgin olive oil

Directions

Keto Diet Breakfast Recipes

1. Add oil to a small skillet and sauté the onion for around 5 minutes. Once tender, remove from the skillet and set aside.

2. Using some non-stick cooking spray, coat a slow cooker and set it aside.

3. Then mix together ¾ cup of cheese, sautéed onion and the rest of the ingredients. Whisk to combine and transfer to the Crockpot.

4. Now sprinkle with the remaining mozzarella on top of the mixture. Cook the contents on low for 1 hour to 1 ½ hours while covered.

5. As soon as the eggs are set, remove from the cooker and serve.

Calories: 139, Carbs 4g, Protein 12g, Fat 8g

Shakshouka Skillet

Prep Time: 10 minutes

Cook Time: 20 minutes

Total Time: 30 minutes

Serves 6

Ingredients

1/2 teaspoon ground cumin

1/4 cup chopped fresh mint leaves

Extra-virgin olive oil

1/2 cup homemade tomato sauce

6 Vine-ripe chopped tomatoes

1/4 cup chopped fresh parsley leaves

6 eggs

1 teaspoon sweet paprika

1 teaspoon salt and pepper

1 teaspoon ground coriander

2 garlic cloves, peeled, chopped

2 green peppers, chopped

1 large yellow onion, chopped

Pinch red pepper flakes, optional

Directions

1. In a skillet, heat olive oil over medium heat and then stir in green peppers, garlic, salt, pepper, spices and onions.

2. Cook and stir the veggies for around 10 minutes or until softened and until the onion is translucent.

3. Then in a bowl, mix together tomato sauce and tomatoes. Pour the mixture into a skillet, and stir to incorporate the ingredients.

4. Now simmer the mixture while uncovered for about 10 to 12 minutes, or until tomato juice is cooked of. Taste and adjust the seasonings, as you would like.

5. Into the tomato mixture, make 6 well-spaced indentations for the eggs and then crack the eggs into the "wells".

6. At this point, lower the heat and then let the eggs cook while covered for another 5 minutes or so.

7. Once the eggs are set, uncover, add in mint and fresh parsley. Season the shakshuka with crushed red pepper or black pepper if you like it.

8. You can serve with a Keto-friendly bread (breads in a later chapter) of choice if you like it.

Calories 192, Carbs 11.8g, Protein 10g, Fat 8.7g

Spicy Veggie Omelet

Prep Time: 10 minutes

Cook Time: 10 minutes

Total Time: 20 minutes

Serves 1 omelet

Ingredients

5 egg whites

1 large egg

1 ounce mozzarella cheese

2 cups baby spinach, organic

4 onions, raw, medium, sliced

Directions

1. Preheat a pan or skillet.

2. Then combine 5 egg whites with 1 egg, stir to mix, and then pour into a pan.

3. Now cook until set on one side while at the same time measuring the onions, cheese and spinach.

4. Flip over the egg mixture; add the onions, cheese and spinach on the top, and then fold. Serve and enjoy the tortilla!

Calories: 266.3, Carbs: 11.3g, Protein: 29.6g, Fat: 9.1g

Chive and Cream Cheese Omelet

Prep Time: 10 minutes

Cook Time: 15 minutes

Total Time: 25 minutes

Serves 2

Ingredients

4 eggs

1 tablespoon olive oil

2 tablespoons water

2 tablespoons minced chives

1/8 teaspoon pepper

1/8 teaspoon salt

Salsa

2 ounces cream cheese, cubed

Directions

1. Heat the oil in a large nonstick skillet over medium-high heat.

2. Then whisk together the chives, eggs, water, salt and pepper, and now add the mixture to the skillet.

3. Cook the mixture until almost set, while pushing the cooked edges to the center.

4. At this point, sprinkle cream cheese on top, and then fold over the filling.

5. Finally put in a plate and slice into two, and then serve with salsa.

305 calories, Carbs 2g, Protein 15g, Fat 27g

Cheesy Italian Omelet

Prep time: 5

Cooking Time: 10 minutes

Total time: 15 minutes

Serves 1

Ingredients

2 oz. fresh mozzarella cheese

5 thin slices fresh, ripe tomato

6 fresh basil leaves

3 thin slices deli Sopressata, salami or prosciutto

1 tablespoon butter

1 tablespoon water

2 eggs

Salt and pepper to taste

Directions

1. In a small bowl, whisk the eggs along with water. Then melt butter in a sauté pan over medium heat.

2. Pour the egg and water mixture in the pan and cook for a few seconds. Now spread the sliced meat on half of the egg mixture.

3. Top with tomatoes, cheese and basil slices, and season with pepper and salt.

4. Now cook the ingredients until half of the egg mixture is firm to be folded over the ingredients, or for around 2 minutes.

5. Using a spatula, gently fold the omelet in half, cover the pan and now cook on low heat for 1 to 2 minutes.

6. As soon as no raw egg is left at the center, tilt the pan and slide the omelet onto a plate. Serve.

451 calories, 36 g fat, 3 g carbs, 33 g protein

Baked Eggs in Portobello Mushroom Caps

Prep Time: 15 minutes

Cook Time: 30 minutes

Total Time: 45 minutes

Serves 4

Ingredients

A little amount of olive oil

1 teaspoon fresh parsley or thyme

¼ teaspoon black pepper

6 slices of prosciutto

6 Portobello mushroom caps

6 farm fresh eggs

Directions

1. Using a dump cloth, clean the mushroom caps and then discard the stems. Scrap out the gills to create a well for the eggs.

2. Season the outsides of your mushroom with some olive oil to prevent it from sticking to the pan. Then arrange the Portobello caps on a baking sheet.

3. Now put a slice of a prosciutto in the mushroom cap and then slide in a cracked egg inside the prosciutto-filled mushroom cap.

4. Season with herbs such as thyme or parsley and some pepper and now put the contents on a baking pan.

5. At this point, cook in a preheated oven at 375 degrees F for around 20 to 30 minutes.

Calories 187, Carbs 4.46g, Protein 11.8g, Fat 13.5g

Baked Star Squash & Eggs

Prep Time: 10 minutes

Cook Time: 30 minutes

Total Time: 40 minutes

Serves 1

Ingredients

1 small to medium egg

1/4 teaspoon dried thyme

1 tablespoon fresh, chopped flat leaf parsley

1 star squash (patty pan)

Directions

1. Remove the tops from your squashes and hollow out a bit of the insides to create rooms for egg and spices.

2. Sprinkle with dried thyme and parsley. Now crack the egg and add it to the squash.

3. Bake at 350 degrees F until the eggs are set, in about 30 to 40 minutes.

Calories 89, Carbs 7g, Proteins 7.5g, Fat 4g

Heirloom Tomato and Swiss chard Eggs Benedict

Prep Time: 15 minutes

Cook Time: 15 minutes

Total Time: 30 minutes

Servings: 4

Ingredients

Blender Hollandaise

1/8 teaspoon cayenne pepper

1-3 teaspoons lemon juice, 15 ml

4 ounces salted butter or ghee

3 large egg yolks

For Swiss chard Eggs Benedict

Salt and pepper

4 large eggs poached

8 ounces Heirloom tomato slices, 4 thick slices

2 cloves of garlic sliced

8 ounces Swiss chard, 200 g

1/2-1 teaspoon of the lemon zest

Garnish

Black pepper cayenne or paprika

Chives green onion, or chopped fresh herbs

Directions

1. Start by making the Blender Hollandaise in the blender. Just add in the egg yolks to the blender, then place the top onto the blender but remove the middle piece. Meanwhile preheat a frying pan over medium heat, and add butter to the pan until melted. Continue to heat until foaming stops. Now turn the blender to low and pour in the hot butter in slowly until the Hollandaise starts to emulsify. Add in the lemon and some pepper then set the blender to high speed. Keep scrapping the sides of the blender and the middle back to the top of the lid. Leave the mixture in the blender to keep it warm until about to serve. Put back the butter-coated pan to the heat.

2. Start preparing the Swiss chard.

Wash the chard, discard the ribs then cut into 2 inch pieces. Then slice the garlic and set aside. Put the frying pan over medium heat until hot, and add in garlic. Cook until fragrant and begins to soften, and then add the cleaned Swiss chard. Cook the chard until it has wilted then season with salt and pepper. Once done with cooking, cover the lid to keep warm and then turn off the heat.

3. Begin making the poached eggs. Fill a frying pan with water to three-quarter full then add a teaspoon of salt and

two teaspoons of vinegar. Set the heat to medium high and heat until it starts to simmer slowly. Then lower the heat the medium. At this point, crack the eggs one by one then carefully open them into the almost simmering water. Keep an eye on the heat under the pan not to allow the water to boil. Cook the cracked eggs for a minute or so then loosen them from the bottom of the pan using a spatula to make them float freely. Poach them for another minute, and then roll them over using a slotted spoon. Then poach for another 2 minutes before removing them from the pan and draining on paper towels.

4. Time to assemble. Just slice the tomato slices about 2 inches long and put them on serving plate. Season the slices with salt and pepper.

5. Divide the chard into various serving plates and then arrange the tomato slices. Add in the eggs, salt, pepper and other seasonings.

6. Add in the Blender Hollandaise and then garnish with your preferred toppings. Serve and enjoy.

Calories 377, Carbs 6g, Protein 10g, Fat 35g

Breakfast Casseroles

Savory Breakfast Casserole

Prep Time: 15 minutes

Cook Time: 30 minutes

Total Time: 45 minutes

Serves 6-9

Ingredients

1/2 yellow onion, diced

1 teaspoon garlic powder

1 teaspoon salt

1 teaspoon onion powder

1 sweet potato, shredded

12 eggs, whisked

1 lb. chorizo, cooked and diced

2 tablespoons hot sauce

1 teaspoon pepper

Directions

1. Preheat an oven to 375 degrees F. Then heat a skillet and then add chorizo. Allow to cook until it starts to crumble.

2. As the chorizo cooks, shred the sweet potato in a food processor and dice the onion.

3. Then beat the eggs into a bowl and add the onion, cooked meat and sweet potato to the bowl. Add other ingredients and combine well.

4. At this point, grease a glass dish and add the egg-meat mixture. Cook until the eggs aren't runny, about 25-30 minutes. You should cook the middle for longer, as it takes time to be completely done.

5. As soon as its set, let sit for 10 minutes before serving.

Calories 316, Carbs 4g, Protein 25g, Fat 34g

Keto Diet Breakfast Recipes

Yellow Squash Casserole

Prep Time: 15 minutes

Cook Time: 30 minutes

Total Time: 45 minutes

Serves 10

Ingredients

1/4 cup butter, melted

1 cup shredded Cheddar cheese

4 cups sliced yellow squash

35 buttery round crackers, crushed

2 eggs, beaten

3/4 cup milk

Black pepper, ground to taste

1 teaspoon salt

2 tablespoons butter

1/2 cup chopped onion

Directions

1. First heat the oven to 400 degrees F. Meanwhile, add onion and squash to a large skillet then pour in some water.

2. Over medium heat, cook the mixture for about 5 minutes, covered. As soon as the squash is tender, drain the mixture and set in a large bowl.

3. Then combine cheese and crackers in a medium bowl and then stir half of the cracker mixture into the onion and squash mixture.

4. Now combine milk and eggs in a small bowl and then add it into the squash-cracker mixture.

5. Then stir in the melted butter and season with some pepper and salt. Spread the mixture into a baking dish (approx. 9x13 inches) and then sprinkle with cracker mixture.

6. At this point, sprinkle the reserved cracker mixture and dot the dish with 2 tablespoons of butter.

7. Bake the casserole batter for 25 minutes or until lightly browned.

Calories 196, Carbs 10.3g, Protein 6.1g, Fat 14.8g

Crock Pot Mexican Breakfast Casserole

Prep Time: 15 minutes

Cook Time: 2 hours 30 minutes

Total Time: 2 hours 45 minutes

Serves 10

Ingredients

1 cup Pepper Jack cheese

1 cup milk

10 eggs

1 cup salsa

1/4 teaspoon pepper

1/4 teaspoon salt

1 teaspoon cumin

1/2 teaspoon coriander

1/2 teaspoon garlic powder

1 teaspoon chili powder

12 ounces Jones Dairy Farm Pork Sausage Roll

Avocado salsa, sour cream, cilantro, optional

Directions

Keto Diet Breakfast Recipes

1. First cook the pork sausage in a large skillet over medium heat until it is no longer pink.

2. Season and add salsa then set aside to slightly cool down.

3. In a separate bowl, whisk the coconut milk with eggs then add in pork to the eggs.

4. Now add in Jack cheese and stir to blend. Grease the bottom of a slow cooker and pour in the egg mixture.

5. Finally cook on low for 5 hours or high for 2 ½ hours. Serve topped with preferred toppings.

Calories 320, Carbs 5.2g, Protein 17.9g, Fat 24.1g

Crockpot Breakfast Casserole

Prep Time: 15 minutes

Cook Time: 4 hours

Total Time: 4 hours 15 minutes

Serves: 8

Ingredients

6 oz. cheddar cheese

1 small head of broccoli, chopped

2 bell peppers, chopped

1/2 onion, chopped

4 strips cooked bacon, optional

30 oz. rutabagas or frozen hash browns

1/2 teaspoon pepper

1 teaspoon salt

1/2 teaspoon garlic salt

2 teaspoons stone mustard, ground

3/4 cup coconut milk

4 egg whites

8 eggs

Directions

1. Whisk together whole eggs, milk, egg whites, garlic, mustard, salt and pepper in a medium bowl and set aside.

2. Grease your slow cooker with oil then put half of the hash browns on the bottom.

3. Then layer half amounts of each of the following: bacon, bell peppers, chopped onion, broccoli and cheese.

4. Add in the rest of the hash browns, top with the remaining veggies, bacon and the cheese. Then pour the egg mixture on top.

5. Then cover the cooker and let cook for 4 hours on low heat. Serve it while hot.

Calories 187.4, Carbs 6.7g, Protein 13.7g, Fat 11.9g

Sausage and Asparagus Casserole

Prep Time: 10 minutes

Cook Time: 40 minutes

Total Time: 50 minutes

Serves: 4-6

Ingredients

Butter or coconut oil

Salt and pepper, to taste

¼ teaspoon garlic powder

1 tablespoon fresh dill, minced

¼ cup coconut milk

8 eggs, whisked

6-8 stalks of asparagus, chopped

1 medium white leek, thinly sliced

1 pound breakfast sausage

Directions

1. Preheat your oven to 325 degrees F. Meanwhile, grease an 8×8 baking pan.

2. In a sauté pan, heat the breakfast sausage over medium heat and then break it into small pieces.

3. When cooked half-way, add in asparagus and leak, only the white part. Cook the mixture until no longer pink.

4. Once ready, remove from heat and drain off excess fat from the pan.

5. Now whisk together pepper, salt, garlic powder, dill, cream and eggs in a medium bowl.

6. Then transfer this mixture to the greased 8×8 baking pan and then add in the sausage mixture. Combine the contents completely.

7. At this point, bake the mixture into the preheated oven for about 35-40. When done, the eggs should be cooked through in the center and firm.

Calories 450, Carbs 14g, Protein 30g, Fat 32.2g

Easy Breakfast Casserole

Prep Time: 15 minutes

Cook Time: 55 minutes

Total Time: 1 hour 10 minutes

Serves: 5-6

Ingredients

½ teaspoon garlic powder

½ teaspoon sea salt

10 free-range eggs, whisked

2 cups spinach, chopped

½ yellow onion, diced

1½ pounds breakfast sausage

½ teaspoon fine sea salt

1 sweet potato, diced

2 tablespoons coconut oil or butter or ghee, melted

Directions

1. First pre-heat your oven to 400 degrees F as you grease a 9x12 baking dish.

2. Then toss diced sweet potatoes in the oil and then sprinkle sea salt.

3. Put the sweet potatoes onto the baking sheet and then bake for around 20-25 minutes, to softness.

4. As your sweet potatoes cook, put a big sauté pan over medium heat and then add in breakfast sausage together with yellow onion. Continue to cook until all the pink color from the sausage disappears.

5. Put your mixture containing the meat into the baking dish and then add in spinach, sweet potatoes and eggs, together with sea salt and garlic powder until fully blended.

6. Finally place over the oven and bake for around 25-30 minutes to have the eggs get set in the middle.

Calories 662, Carbs 12g, Protein 40.4g, Fat 50g

Breakfast Mock Casserole

Prep Time: 15 minutes

Cook Time: 1 hour 15 minutes

Total Time: 1 hour 30 minutes

Serves 8

Ingredients

1/4 teaspoon sage

1/2 teaspoon garlic powder

1/2 teaspoon onion powder

Salt and pepper to taste

4 tablespoon butter

6 tablespoon maple syrup

4 oz. cheddar cheese

10 large eggs

1 lb. breakfast sausage

1/4 cup flaxseed meal

1 cup almond flour

Directions

1. Preheat your oven to 350 degrees. Meanwhile over medium, place a pan on the stove and then add the sausage. Break it up using a wooden spoon and cook until browned.

2. Combine the dry ingredients in a bowl and the wet ingredients in a separate bowl. Mix them together.

3. Add 4 tablespoons of the syrup and mix well to blend. Then add the cheese to the ingredients and continue to mix.

4. As soon as the sausage has browned and is crispy, add all the ingredients into the mixture along with the excess fats. Mix again to blend.

5. At this point, line a 9×9 casserole dish using a parchment paper then pour the mixture into it.

6. Drizzle the casserole with 2 tablespoon of the remaining syrup to add flavor. Put the casserole in the oven and bake until cooked through, in about 45 to 55 minutes.

7. Now remove the oven and let it cool for a moment. Then hold the edges of the casserole with parchment paper and lift out the baked dish.

8. Slice and serve the casserole, preferably drizzled with additional syrup, or sugar-free ketchup.

Calories 447, Carbs 5.17g, Protein 26g, Fats 36g

Keto Diet Breakfast Recipes

Egg Casserole with Sausage and Cheese

Prep Time: 20 minutes

Cook Time: 2 hours 20 minutes

Total Time: 2 hours 40 minutes

Serves 10

Ingredients

14 eggs, beaten until well-combined

Black pepper, fresh ground

1-2 teaspoons Spike Seasoning

½ cup sliced green onions

2 tablespoons onions for garnish

2 cups grated cheddar cheese

1 green pepper, diced

24 oz. breakfast sausage links

1 ½ cups cottage cheese, rinsed and drained

3 teaspoons olive oil, divided

Directions

1. Grease a crockpot with non-stick spray or olive oil. Then place cottage cheese into a fine mesh colander. Put the

cheese in the sink and rinse with water to wash away the creamy part.

2. In a frying pan, heat a teaspoon of olive oil over medium high heat and cook half of the sausage links until fully browned. Transfer the sausage onto a cutting board to cool down.

3. Now heat a teaspoon of oil and cool the remaining half of the sausage and move it to the cutting board too. You can cook the sausages altogether if your pan can accommodate them.

4. Heat a teaspoon of oil and brown the pepper pieces for about 2 or 3 minutes. You can cook them directly if you want them somehow crunchy.

5. Once done, cut the sausage links into halves and layer them in the crockpot along with diced or stripped green peppers.

6. Season with cottage cheese and then with the grated cheddar cheese. Top the mixture with sliced onions and top with black pepper and spike seasoning.

7. At this point, beat the eggs until well incorporated and then pour over the cut sausages, cheese and cottage cheese. Distribute the peppers and sausages in the cooking pot using a fork.

8. Close the lid in place and cook the mixture on low heat for 2 hours or more until the cheese is well melted and the eggs are firm in the center.

9. Finally top with sliced green onions and enjoy the breakfast hot!

Calories 403, Carbs 3.6g, Protein 27.2g, Fat 30.0g

Overnight Breakfast Casserole

Prep Time: 15 minutes

Cook Time: 6 hours 15 minutes

Total Time: 6 hours 30 minutes

Serves 10

Ingredients

1/4 teaspoon cracked black pepper

3/4 teaspoon dry mustard

1 teaspoon sea salt

1/4 cup full-fat coconut milk

1/2 cup almond milk

16 large eggs, beaten

1 orange bell pepper, seeded and diced

1 red bell pepper, seeded and diced

1 pound sweet potato, peeled and shredded

1/2 cup yellow onion, diced

6 ounces bacon, chopped

1/2 pound bulk breakfast sausage, crumbled

Softened ghee, to greasing the crockpot

Green onions, for garnish

Directions

1. First grease the bottom and sides of a crockpot using softened ghee or palm shortening.

2. Then cook the onion, bacon and the sausage in the slow cooker until the onion is softened and the sausage browned, or for about 10 to 12 minutes.

3. Discard any excess fat. Now add in shredded sweet potato in the crockpot and press them down gently.

4. Add in the onion and meat mixture and bell peppers on top.

5. In a separate bowl, whisk together eggs, mustard, salt, milk and pepper. Pour into the crockpot.

6. Cook the mixture on low for 6 to 8 hours or until cooked through.

Calories 267, Carbs 7.5g, Protein 11.3g, Fat 18.7g

Instant Pot Recipes

Breakfast Sandwich

Prep Time: 15 minutes

Cook Time: 15 minutes

Total Time: 30 minutes

Serves 4

Ingredients

8 slices gluten-free bread

4 tablespoon cheddar cheese, grated

4 eggs

4 prosciutto, thinly sliced

1/4 teaspoon olive oil

4 cups water

Directions

1. To an Instant Pot, add a cup of water and then put into a steamer tray or trivet.

2. Into the bottom of the ramekin, place little amount of coconut oil, butter, or olive oil and evenly coat its insides.

3. Now into the bottom of the ramekin, put a slice of prosciutto and then add in the egg white or egg substitute.

Follow this with cracked pepper and then sprinkle shredded cheese on top.

4. Use a piece of tin foil to cover the ramekin, and set it into the steamer basket. Now insert the basket into the cooker's pot just on top of the trivet.

5. Close the cooker and lock the lid in place, then cook on low pressure for 6 minutes.

6. Once ready, release the pressure naturally for around 5 minutes.

7. Meanwhile, toast up the rye bread slices. Once cool, open the pressure cooker and lift out the steamer basket.

8. Now remove the ramekin and run a butter knife through the edge of the egg creation. Tip it out and set onto the slice of rye. Serve it immediately.

Calories: 321, Carbs: 11g, Protein 6.8g, Fat 3g

Egg Muffins in the Pressure Cooker

Prep Time: 15 minutes

Cook Time: 15 minutes

Total Time: 30 minutes

Serves 2

Ingredients

1/4 teaspoon lemon pepper

4 slices precooked bacon, crumbled

1 green onion, diced

4 eggs

4 tablespoons nutritional yeast

Directions

1. Place the steamer basket in Instant Pot then add 1 ½ cups of water.

2. Break the eggs into a measuring bowl and then add in lemon pepper. Now divide nutritional yeast over 4 silicon muffin cups.

3. Pour the beaten egg mixture into each cup and combine using a fork.

4. At this point, put the muffin cups into the basket and lock the lid. Cook for 8 minutes at high pressure.

5. Then turn off the Instant Pot, wait for 2-3 minutes then quick release pressure.

6. Open the lid, remove the steamer basket and lift the muffin cups. Serve and enjoy.

Calories 542, Carbs 6.5g, Protein 29g, Fat 43.8g

Keto Friendly Cornish Hens

Prep Time: 10 minutes

Cook Time: 10 minutes

Total Time: 20 minutes

Serves 2

Ingredients

1 1/2 cup water

2 teaspoons Worcestershire sauce, soy free

2 stalks celery, chopped

2 bay leaves

4 cloves garlic, chopped

2 onions chopped

Salt and pepper

2 tablespoons oil

2 Cornish hens

Directions

1. In an Instant Pot, add the oil followed by the brown hens.

2. Use pepper and salt to season the chicken and add the remaining ingredients. Then pour over the chicken.

3. Seal the cooker and heat under low heat for 8 minutes, ensuring the pressure regulator rocks slowly.

4. Remove the contents from the heat and allow the pressure to drop naturally.

Calories 472, Carbs 16.8g, Protein 50g, Fat 21.9g

Eggs en Cocotte in the Instant Pot

Prep Time: 2 minutes

Cook Time: 3 minutes

Total Time: 5 minutes

Serves: 3

Ingredients

1 cup water

Pepper, freshly ground

Sea salt

1 tablespoon chives

3 fresh pasture raised eggs

3 tablespoons cream

Butter, room temp

Directions

1. Coat the ramekins with butter then add a tablespoon of cream into each.

2. Crack an egg into each ramekin taking care not to break the yolks.

3. Sprinkle the eggs with chives, and put the rack into the cooking pot. Add 1 cup of water to the Instant Pot and put the ramekins on the rack.

4. Lock the Instant Pot and cook for 2 minutes. After timer goes off, switch and quick release the pressure.

5. Using kitchen towel or hot pad, remove the ramekins from cooking pot.

6. Season with pepper and salt. Serve on toast.

Calories 120g, Carbs 0.9g, Protein 3.7g, Fat 11.2g

Crust-less Meat Lovers Quiche

Prep Time: 10 minutes

Cook Time: 40 minutes

Total Time: 50 minutes

Serves 4

Ingredients

1 cup cheese

2 large green onions, chopped

1/2 cup diced ham

1 cup ground sausage, cooked

4 slices bacon, cooked and crumbled

1/8 teaspoon black pepper, ground

1/4 teaspoon salt

1/2 cup almond or coconut milk

6 large eggs, beaten

Directions

1. Add 1 ½ cups of water into metal trivet of Instant Pot.

2. Whisk together milk, eggs, salt and pepper into a large bowl. Then add in ham, sausage, bacon, non-dairy cheese and green onions to a 1 quart soufflé dish and combine them.

3. Now pour the egg mixture over the meat, and stir to incorporate them. With aluminum foil, loosely cover the soufflé dish.

4. Drop the dish into the trivet of the cooking pot using an aluminum sling. Lock the lid and cook for 30 minutes at high pressure.

5. Once cooked, turn off; allow to cool for 10 minutes then quick release. Open the lid and remove the foil.

6. Serve. You can sprinkle some additional cheese then broil to melt and lightly brown.

Calories 448, Carbs 15.6g, Proteins 26.9g, Fat 31g

Pressure Cooker Banana Bread

Prep Time: 20 minutes

Cook Time: 55 minutes

Total Time: 1 hour 15 minutes

Serves 12

Ingredients

1 1/2 teaspoon cream of tartar

1/3 cup coconut/almond milk

Pinch of salt

1/2 teaspoon baking soda

1 teaspoon baking powder

1 1/2 cup cassava flour

2 mashed, ripe bananas

1 teaspoon vanilla

1 egg

3/4 cup coconut sugar

1/3 cup softened ghee

Directions

Keto Diet Breakfast Recipes

1. In a small bowl, add coconut, almond or cashew milk and cream of tartar. Set it aside.

2. Cream together coconut sugar and butter, then add in vanilla and eggs. Mix well to incorporate. Add mashed bananas and mix well.

3. Now mix cassava flour, baking soda, baking powder and salt and slowly add to the eggs mixture. Then add in buttermilk mixture and stir.

4. Using foil that is sprayed with cooking spray, cover the batter to ensure it doesn't stick.

5. Add the mixture to a greased 7 inch pan. Then add in 2 cups of water into the cooking pot of Instant Pot. Put the metal trivet rack in the bottom of cooking pot.

6. Carefully lower the pan with batter onto the trivet. Then close the lid and seal it by moving the knob on top.

7. Set to Manual function for 30 minutes. Let the Instant Pot come to pressure and bake the ingredients.

8. Soon after the pressure cooker beeps, let it naturally release pressure for about 15-20 minutes. Then carefully remove the lid after pressure drops.

9. Remove the trivet and the pan, along with the foil. Let the bread cool onto a wire rack in the pan. Don't remove from the pan yet.

10. Once cool completely, store in the fridge preferably overnight to take in the morning with coffee.

Keto Diet Breakfast Recipes

Calories 145, Carbs 15g, Protein 1.7g, Fat 8.9g

Note about the banana: I know you know that bananas are not exactly Ketogenic diet friendly, as they tend to be very high in carb i.e. 25g per average sized banana. Don't worry though given that you won't be eating the 2 bananas at once- the recipe serves 12, which means your carb intake won't be too high. Nonetheless, it is still best to prepare this recipe and use it just before workouts or after workouts.

Instant Pot Mug Cakes

Prep Time: 5 minutes

Cook Time: 10 minutes

Total Time: 15 minutes

Serves 1

Ingredients

1/8 teaspoon salt

1/2 teaspoon vanilla

1 tablespoon maple syrup

1 egg

1/3 cup almond flour

Directions

1. In a small bowl, mix together almond floor with other ingredients.

2. Spray with oil and then scoop the mixture into an 8 ounce mason jar.

3. Put a trivet in the instant pot's bowl and add a cup of water. Use foil to cover the mug cake jars and put into the trivet.

4. Inspect the sealing ring, close the lid and secure the pressure valve.

5. Set the pressure cooker to "manual" and cook time to 10 minutes. Then quick release the pressure by opening the steam release valve.

6. Using tongs remove the mason jars and set them onto a cooling rack. You can serve either cold or warm.

Calories 190, Carbs 14.7g, Protein 9g, Fat 9.8g

Korean Style Steamed Eggs

Prep Time: 5 minutes

Cook Time: 5 minutes

Total Time: 10 minutes

Serves 1

Ingredients

Chopped scallions

Garlic powder

Salt

Pepper

Sesame seeds

⅓ cup cold water

1 large egg

Directions

1. In a small bowl, mix together the egg and water. Once done, strain the egg mixture into heat-proof bowl over a fine strainer.

2. Add in the other ingredients and combine well; then set aside.

3. Now add in a cup of water into the inner pot of an Instant Pot; and place the steamer basket or trivet in the pot.

4. Place the bowl that has the egg mixture on the steamer basket and then close the lid tight; along with the vent valve.

5. Now set the cooker to manual setting on "High" and set the duration to 5 minutes.

6. Once ready, the timer should go off. Quick release, open the cooker and serve.

Calories 82, Carbs 3.2g, Protein 3.7g, Fat 6.2g

Breakfast Salads & Side Dishes

Breakfast Spinach Salad

Prep Time: 15 minutes

Cook Time: 15 minutes

Total Time: 30 minutes

Serves 4

Ingredients

1/2 cup vegetable oil

1/4 teaspoon ground black pepper

1/2 teaspoon celery seeds

1/2 teaspoon salt

1/2 onion, chopped

3 eggs

1/4 pound bacon

1 pound spinach, rinsed and chopped

1 1/3 ounces croutons (Keto bread)

2 tablespoons sliced fresh mushrooms

2 1/2 tablespoons cider vinegar

1 1/2 teaspoons Dijon Mustard

5 1/2 tablespoons Splenda

Directions

1. Put eggs in a saucepan and then add in cold water to completely cover them. Bring the water (along with the eggs) to a boil.

2. Cover and then remove the eggs from heat. Let stand in hot water for about 10 minutes.

3. Remove the eggs from water, cool for few minutes and then peel and chop them.

4. At this point, drain the bacon into a large and deep skillet, and then cook it over high heat until it turns evenly brown. Drain the bacon, crumble and set it aside.

5. Now make the dressing by mixing vinegar, sugar, onion, pepper, salt, Dijon Mustard and celery seed into a blender. Process the mixture until smooth.

6. In a large salad bowl, mix together bacon, mushrooms, croutons and eggs then toss evenly.

7. Drizzle the dressing over the salad to lightly coat, toss and then serve.

Calories 483, Carbs 12g, Protein 27g, Fat 37.3g

Warming Breakfast Salad

Prep Time: 15 minutes

Cook Time: 5 minutes

Total Time: 20 minutes

Serves: 1

Ingredients

2 slices extra lean ham

2 medium tomatoes

1 medium egg

150g baby leaf spinach

Directions

1. Start by rinsing the spinach and then let it dry.

2. Turn on your grill and add water to a pan over medium heat. Bring the water to a boil, and poach an egg.

3. Slice your tomatoes in half and put them under the grill, and proceed to slice the ham as the tomatoes and eggs continue to cook.

4. Now layer the spinach leaves onto a plate and then sprinkle the chopped ham on the veggies.

5. Put the cooked tomato and egg on to the bed of spinach to serve.

Keto Diet Breakfast Recipes

Calories: 159, Carbs 9.8g, Protein 15.9g, Fats 6.8g

Canadian Bacon & Asparagus Salad

Prep Time: 15 minutes

Cook Time: 0 minutes

Total Time: 15 minutes

Serves 6

Ingredients

For the Dressing:

1/2 teaspoon mixed herbs: dill, chervil or tarragon

1/4 teaspoon pepper

1/2 teaspoon salt

1 lemon, juiced

1 tablespoon Dijon mustard

1/4 cup olive oil

For the Salad

1 shallot, finely sliced, sautéed until crisp in oil

1 avocado, sliced

2 large eggs, soft or hard boiled and peeled

1 teaspoon olive oil

6 ounces Jones Canadian Bacon, julienned

1 small bunch asparagus, cooked

5 ounces arugula, washed and dried

Directions

1. To make the salad dressing, put all the ingredients in a small jar that has a tight fitting lid. Shake the mixture until the contents have emulsified.

2. To make the salad, simply toss the dressing, asparagus and the salad greens together.

3. Put each halve of the mixture on a different serving plate.

4. Now in a skillet and over medium heat, sauté the bacon until lightly browned. Put on the salad along with the sliced avocado.

5. Garnish the breakfast salad with crispy shallots.

Calories 229, Carbs 9g, Protein 9.9g, Fat 18g

Lemon Garlic Mushrooms salad

Prep Time: 5 minutes

Cook Time: 10 minutes

Total Time: 15 minutes

Serves 2-3

Ingredients

1-2 tablespoons lemon juice

A pinch of black pepper

½ teaspoon sea salt

1 tablespoon coconut oil or olive oil

Zest of ½ lemon

2 garlic cloves, peeled and diced

5 springs of fresh thyme, leaves only

10-11oz sliced button mushrooms

Cracked black pepper, to taste

Directions

1. In a large frying pan, heat some ghee until hot and then add in thyme and mushrooms.

2. Cook the mixture on high until browned or for about 3 to 4 minutes, and then lower the heat to medium.

3. Flip the mushrooms over as soon as they start to release a liquid and cook the other side for around 2 minutes.

4. Then add in thyme, garlic, pepper, butter, lemon zest and sea salt and cook for about 1-2 minutes, while stirring.

4. At this point, drizzle with some fresh lemon juice, toss a little to incorporate together and then serve.

Calories 96, Carbs 5g, Protein 0,85g, Fat 8.9g

Greek Salad

Prep Time: 5 minutes

Cook Time: 0 minutes

Total Time: 5 minutes

Serves: 2

Ingredients

Salt and pepper to taste

Sprinkle oregano

Drizzle balsamic vinegar

Drizzle olive oil

30g good quality feta, chopped or crumbled

¼ red onion, sliced

1 Lebanese cucumber, chopped

¼ capsicum, chopped

1 large tomato or 2 smaller tomatoes, diced

Directions

1. In a bowl, add in all the listed ingredients while using tongs to blend them together.

2. When well combined, pour onto 2 cups and then serve with grilled beef, chicken or fish if you like it.

Keto Diet Breakfast Recipes

Calories 118, Carbs 4.1g, Protein 4.1g, Fat 8.9g

Greek Beef Salad

Prep Time: 10 minutes

Cook Time: 15 minutes

Total Time: 25 minutes

Serves 2

Ingredients

Sprinkle of oregano

1 chili, deseeded and sliced

2 handfuls lettuce

1 small cucumber, sliced

1 tablespoon crumbled feta, good quality

4 cup mushroom, sliced

2 cloves garlic, crushed

½ lemon, juiced

1 tablespoon olive oil

6 cherry tomatoes

300g Rump Steak, fully trimmed of fat

Directions

1. On your steak, drizzle a teaspoon of olive oil, and then rub a small sprinkle of oregano and a clove of crushed garlic.

2. Season the steak with some salt and pepper. Then heat a griddle pan or a BBQ pan on high heat, for about 5 minutes.

3. At this point, cook the steak on the hot pan for about 3-4 minutes on each side.

4. Then into a bowl, assemble the salad ingredients and then drizzle sliced chili, squeeze of lemon, sprinkle of oregano, clove of crushed garlic and remaining olive oil.

5. You can use tongs to ensure that the ingredients are fully coated. Then remove the beef from heat and put onto a plate.

6. Allow the cooked meat to rest while covered with foil, for 5 minutes. Finally slice into strips before serving.

Calories 363, Carbs 2.2g, Protein 50.6g, Fat 16.2g

Artichoke, Edamame, and Asparagus Salad

Prep Time: 10 minutes

Cook Time: 5 minutes

Total Time: 15 minutes

Serves: 4

Ingredients

1 ounce shaved Parmesan cheese

1 pound medium asparagus, cut into thirds

1 cup frozen green soybeans (edamame)

1 (14-ounce) can artichoke hearts, quartered

1/4 teaspoon pepper

1/4 teaspoon salt

1/2 teaspoon dried oregano

1 tablespoon lemon juice, fresh

2 tablespoons extra-virgin olive oil

1 garlic clove, peeled and halved lengthwise

Directions

1. Coat the insides of a salad bowl with garlic clove. Throw away the garlic.

2. Then add in pepper, salt, oregano, lemon juice and oil. Whisk the contents completely and then add in artichokes.

3. Toss the mixture slowly and allow to rest for some time at normal root temperature.

4. Put the soybeans in salted water that is boiling, and cook for about 2 minutes.

5. Then add in asparagus that has its tough ends removed, and cut diagonally into thirds.

6. Now cook the soybeans and asparagus for 3 minutes. When crisp tender, rinse under cool water, drain and then blot dry using paper towel.

7. Combine the soybeans and asparagus mixture to the artichoke mixture, and then toss well.

8. At this point, pour the new mixture into 4 individual plates and then arrange shaved Parmesan over each salad to serve.

Calories 184, Carbs 12g, Protein 11g, Fats 10g

A Skinny Caesar

Prep Time: 15 minutes

Cook Time: 12 minutes

Total Time: 27 minutes

Serves 4

Ingredients

1 1/4 cups croutons, fat-free

8 cups romaine lettuce, into 2-inch strips

1/4 cup shaved Parmesan cheese, fresh

2 tablespoons Parmesan cheese, grated

1 tablespoon water

1/2 teaspoon anchovy paste

3/4 teaspoon minced garlic

1 teaspoon Worcestershire sauce

1 1/2 teaspoons red wine vinegar

1 1/2 teaspoons Dijon mustard

1 tablespoon extra-virgin olive oil

2 tablespoons lemon juice, fresh

1/2 cup silken soft tofu

1/4 and 1/8 teaspoon black pepper, divided and freshly ground

1/4 and 1/8 teaspoon kosher salt, divided

1 pound chicken breast halves, skinless and boneless

Olive oil cooking spray

Directions

1. Over medium high heat, grill a pan.

2. Meanwhile, coat the chicken breasts using olive oil spray. Season the misted meat breast with a ¼ teaspoon of pepper and salt.

3. Now grill your chicken until it is cooked through, or for about 5-6 minutes per side.

4. Cool the cooked chicken on a cutting board for about 5 minutes to help in redistribution of juices. When cool, cut your chicken into bite size pieces.

5. Then into a blender, combine the soft tofu, minced garlic, fresh lemon juice, red wine vinegar, extra-virgin olive oil, Dijon mustard, Worcestershire sauce, anchovy paste and then add the remaining pepper and salt.

6. Process the ingredients until fully combined and creamy. If necessary, scrap down the blender sides. To thin the creamy mixture, you can add about a tablespoon of water. Now stir in the grated parmesan.

7. In a large bowl, toss the dressing, lettuce and croutons and then divide the mixture into 4 serving plates.

8. At this point, put the chicken over the salad, and then sprinkle shaved parmesan onto each of the plates.

Calories 269, Carbs 13g, Protein 31g, Fat 10g

Blackened Chicken Salad with Tomato Chutney

Prep Time: 5 minutes

Cook Time: 12 minutes

Total Time: 17 minutes

Serves: 4

Ingredients

1/3 cup olive oil vinaigrette, reduced-fat

1 cup Tomato Chutney

1 cup yellow bell pepper, chopped

1 cup salad cucumber, sliced

1 (10-ounce) package romaine salad greens

Cooking spray

2 teaspoons steak seasoning, blackened

4 (4-ounce) chicken breast halves, skinless, boneless

Directions

1. Start by sprinkling some blackened steak seasoning on the chicken.

2. Then over medium heat, heat a large bon-stick skillet as you coat the chicken using the cooking spray.

3. Add to the pan and cook on both sides until fully cooked, or for about 6 minutes.

4. Into a bowl, mix together salad greens, salad cucumber, yellow bell pepper and olive oil vinaigrette and toss completely.

5. At this point, spoon the greens mixture on 4 individual serving plates and then slice the chicken into thin strips, diagonally.

6. Layer your cooked chicken over the salads and then spoon the chutney over the meat.

Calories 247, Carbs 11.4g, Protein 28.8g, Fat 5.8g

Breads and Pastries

Crockpot Breakfast Meatloaf

Prep Time: 15 minutes

Cook Time: 3 hours 30 minutes

Total Time:3 hours 45 minutes

Serves 8

Ingredients

1 teaspoon sea salt

1 teaspoon paprika

1 teaspoon black pepper

2 teaspoons dried thyme

2 teaspoons ground sage

2 teaspoons red pepper flakes

2 teaspoons dried oregano

2 teaspoons fennel seeds, ground

1 garlic clove

8 tablespoons almond flour

2 eggs

2 lbs. ground pork

2 cups diced onion

1 tablespoon coconut oil

Directions

1. At low medium heat, soften the onion in a tablespoon of oil until transparent. Then remove from heat and let cool.

2. Add all the ingredients to a large bowl apart from the ground pork. Stir or whisk to blend.

3. Add in the softened onions and the ground pork to the bowl and combine the ingredients manually, is using your hands.

4. Then pick the meat mixture and put it in the center of the crockpot's insert. Shape it into a loaf and position it half an inch from the sides of the insert.

5. Once done, pat the top the loaf and close the crockpot's lid. Cook the meatloaf on low for 3 hours, or until the internal temperature is 150 degrees F.

6. Then turn off the crockpot and remove the lid to make it easier to remove the meatloaf. Now let the meatloaf cool for up to 30 minutes and then move it to a separate dish.

7. You can serve immediately or keep it refrigerated overnight and serve for breakfast. To serve, simply reheat the slices at low medium heat for a minute or two.

Calories 412.6, Carbs 5.0g, Protein 32.5g, Fat 28.7g

Keto Mini Meatloaves

Prep Time: 15 minutes

Cook Time: 30 minutes

Total Time: 45 minutes

Serves 6

Ingredients

1/4 teaspoon grated nutmeg

1 teaspoon dried thyme

1 teaspoon garlic powder

2 teaspoons onion powder

2 teaspoons pepper

2 teaspoons salt

1/3 cup coconut flour

4 eggs, lightly beaten

2 carrots, grated or finely diced

6 ounces mushrooms, finely diced

1 medium onion, finely diced

1-2 teaspoons oil

10 ounces frozen, chopped spinach

Keto Diet Breakfast Recipes

2 pounds ground meat –beef or pork

Directions

1. First preheat your oven to 375 degrees F.

2. Then thaw the spinach, squeeze out any extra water and set it aside. Over medium heat, warm a pan then add oil.

3. Once hot, fry the mushrooms and onions until some liquid has cooked out of the mushrooms and the onions are translucent. Set the mixture aside to cool.

4. Now put the ground meat in a large bowl and add in coconut flour, beaten eggs, onion and mushroom mixture, spinach and all the spices. Combine well using your hands.

5. At this point, fill 18 regularly sized muffin pans or tins with the batter. You may need to grease the muffin tins beforehand.

6. Cook the meatloaf until the internal temperature reaches 160 degrees, in about 20 to 30 minutes.

7. Let the meatloaf cool and then loosen it from the sides of the pan using a knife. Serve with marinara sauce that hasn't been artificially sweetened (we prepared this earlier in the book).

Calories 403, Carbs 18g, Protein 37.9g, Fat 20g

Grain-free Blueberry Muffin

Prep Time: 15 minutes

Cook Time: 20 minutes

Total Time: 35 minutes

Serves: 6

Ingredients

¼ cup fresh blueberries

1 egg, room temperature

2 tablespoons coconut oil, melted

½ cup coconut milk, full fat

2 tablespoons raw honey

⅛ Teaspoon baking soda

1 cup blanched almond flour

Pinch of salt

Optional

1/4 cup chopped nuts

1/3 cup of dark chocolate chips

1 teaspoon vanilla extract

Directions

Keto Diet Breakfast Recipes

1. Preheat the oven to about 350 degrees F. Then get a non-stick muffin pan or instead line muffin tin with baking cups.

2. Combine salt, baking soda and almond flour in a bowl and then whisk together egg, coconut oil, coconut milk and honey in a separate bowl.

3. Mix the dry and wet ingredients together using a rubber spatula, taking care not to over mix.

4. Now slowly fold the blueberries to form batter. Spoon the batter into the muffin pan or muffin tin to the top.

5. Bake the contents of the muffin tin for about 20 to 25 minutes. Insert a toothpick into the muffin to test if it comes out clean.

6. Put the pan over a wire rack to cool down and wait for the muffins to cool down.

Calories 1138, Carbs 9.4g, Protein 2g, Fat 11g

Keto Lemon Poppy-seed Muffins

Prep Time: 15 minutes

Cook Time: 30 minutes

Total Time: 45 minutes

Serves 12

Ingredients

25 drops liquid stevia

1 teaspoon vanilla extract

3 tablespoon lemon juice

Zest of 2 lemons

3 large eggs

1/4 cup heavy cream

1/4 cup salted butter, melted

2 tablespoon poppy seeds

1 teaspoon baking powder

1/3 cup erythritol

1/4 cup golden flaxseed meal

3/4 cup blanched almond flour

Directions

Keto Diet Breakfast Recipes

1. First preheat an oven to 350 degrees F; and then combine together poppy seeds, erythritol, flaxseed meal and almond flour using a fork.

2. Then stir in the eggs, melted butter and heavy cream and continue to beat until you obtain a smooth consistency. Make sure that no visible lumps are left in your batter.

3. Now add in vanilla extract, liquid stevia, lemon juice, lemon zest and baking powder and combine fully.

4. Subdivide the batter into 12 equally-sized cupcake molds. You can use ordinary muffin pan or silicon cupcake molds.

5. Then bake the cupcake contents for about 18-20 minutes or until the surface turns somehow brown. You can bake on the higher side in order to achieve a better crust on the bottom.

6. Once done, remove from the oven and let it cool on the counter for about 10 minutes.

7. Finally slice the cakes and serve, preferably with a half pad of butter between the muffins.

Calories 130, Carbs 3.6g, Protein 4g, Fat 11.7g

Bacon cheeseburger Quiche

Prep Time: 30 minutes

Cook Time: 45 minutes

Total Time: 1 hour 15 minutes

Serves 6

Ingredients

8 oz. cheddar or Swiss cheese, shredded

½ cup half and half

½ cup mayonnaise

3 eggs

4 slices cooked bacon, chopped

1 small chopped onion

1 lb. hamburger

Garlic powder, if desired

Directions

1. First brown the hamburger with onion and then mix in bacon. Now press the hamburger-bacon mixture into the bottom of a deep dish pie pan.

2. In a mixer bowl, combine the other ingredients and whip them well.

3. Then pour the mixture over the beef and now bake it until its top is brown and well set. This should take around 40-45 minutes.

3. Once done, cool for about 15-20 minutes and then slice it.

Calories 470, Carbs 4g, Protein 27.5g, Fat 39g

Keto Salmon & Cream Cheese Mug Muffin

Prep Time: 15 minutes

Cook Time: 5 minutes

Total Time: 20 minutes

Serves 2

Ingredients

2 tablespoons water

2 tablespoons cream or coconut milk

1 large egg, free-range or organic

¼ teaspoon baking soda

¼ cup flaxmeal

¼ cup almond flour

Pinch of salt

2 tablespoons spring onion or chives, freshly chopped

60g smoked salmon

2 dollops full-fat sour cream or cream cheese, optional

Directions

1. In a small bowl, put all the ingredients and mix them well.

2. Add in the egg, cream and water and combine with a fork.

3. Finely chop the chives and slice the smoked salmon. Add salmon and chives to the mixture and mix well.

4. Now microwave for 60-90 seconds on high. Then top with cream cheese and serve.

Calories 374, Carbs 9.5 g, Protein 17.2 g, Fat 32.3 g

Low carb Taco Egg Muffins

Prep Time: 15 minutes

Cook Time: 25 minutes

Total Time: 40 minutes

Serves 6

Ingredients

1/2 cup salsa

1/2 cup sour cream

10 black olives, sliced

3 oz. mixed bell peppers, diced

1 cup sharp cheddar cheese, shredded

12 large eggs

2 oz. onion, diced

3 tablespoon Taco Seasoning

8 oz. ground beef

Directions

1. First preheat the oven to 350 degrees F. Then lightly oil a tin or go for a non-stick silicone bake-ware.

2. Over medium high heat, add onions and ground beef in a large skillet and sauté until the meat is browned.

Keto Diet Breakfast Recipes

3. Now drain the grease from the skillet and mix in taco seasoning with about 1/3 cup of water.

4. Lower the heat to low and let the mixture to simmer until thickened, or for around 3 to 4 minutes.

5. Once done, whisk the eggs in a large mixing bowl using a fork, then mix in olives, bell peppers and the cheese.

6. Mix in the beef into the mixture and pour the batter into muffin tin. Finally bake for about 25 minutes.

7. To serve, top each muffin with salsa and sour cream.

Calories 330, Carbs 7.0g, Protein 21g, Fat 17g

Shell Cheese Taco Cups

Prep Time: 15 minutes

Cook Time: 45 minutes

Total Time: 60 minutes

Serves 4

Ingredients

6-8 slices of cheese

Cheese cups

Salsa

3 tablespoons cilantro

Juice from 1 lime

1/2 fresh jalapeno, diced finely

3 tablespoons diced red onion

2 Roma tomatoes, diced

Optional

Avocado

Sour cream

Your preferred taco meat

Directions

Keto Diet Breakfast Recipes

1. First preheat oven to 375 degrees F.

2. Put the sliced cheese on a baking sheet lined with parchment paper leaving a few inches between the slices.

3. Bake until bubbly and begins to brown around the edges or for around 5 minutes.

4. Then remove from the baking sheet and allow to cool for a few minutes.

5. You can now pick up the slices and put them in a muffin tin to create a cup shape, and allow to cool for another 10 minutes.

6. To make the salsa, put the tomatoes, lime juice, jalapeno, onions and cilantro in a medium bowl.

7. Then keep this salsa mixture refrigerated while covered for about 30 minutes.

8. You can also serve immediately if you like it that way though keeping longer in the fridge makes it more flavorful.

Calories 159, Carb 4.7g, Protein 9.6g, Fat 11.6g

Avocado & Bacon Muffins

Prep Time: minutes

Cook Time: minutes

Total Time: minutes

Makes 12

Ingredients

Salt & pepper

1/2 teaspoon baking soda

1/2 cup coconut flour

1 cup coconut milk

2 cups avocado

4 eggs

6 short cut bacon rashers

1 small onion

Directions

1. Preheat the oven to 350 degrees F and then use coconut oil to grease 12 muffin cups.

2. Finely dice the bacon and onion and brown these in a fry pan.

3. Meanwhile, use a fork to mix the eggs and avocado together and then stir in the milk.

4. Then add in salt and pepper, baking soda and coconut floor and mix well to break up all lumps.

5. Now fold through the 3 quarters of the onion and cooked bacon mixture.

6. Then divide the mixture between the 12 muffin cups and top with the reserved onion and bacon.

7. Bake the cups in the preheated oven for about 20 minutes; and cool before you remove the dish from the cups.

8. Serve immediately or alternatively keep chilled in the fridge for outdoor breakfasts.

Calories 108, Carbs 4.5g, Protein 4.5g, Fat 8.3g

Burgers, Sandwiches and Breakfast Meats

Turkey Crusted Crockpot Breakfast

Prep Time: 15 minutes

Cook Time: 15 minutes

Total Time: 30 minutes

Serves 6-8

Ingredients

1 1/2 cups shredded Monterey Jack cheese

1/2 teaspoons pepper

1 cup cottage cheese

6 eggs

1 chopped red bell pepper

1/2 chopped onion

1/2 teaspoons Mrs. Dash

1/2 teaspoons fennel seed

1/2 teaspoons sage

1/2 teaspoons onion powder

1/2 teaspoons garlic powder

1 pound lean ground turkey

½ teaspoon salt

Directions

1. Put the raw turkey meat in the slow cooker and then stir in onion, garlic, fennel, sage and the Mrs. Dash. Stir the ingredients to blend them together.

2. Spread the turkey meat over the bottom of the slow cooker using the back of the spoon.

3. Then chop the veggies and now layer them over the poultry meat. In a medium-sized bowl, whisk the eggs.

4. Then stir in cottage cheese, pepper and salt into the whisked eggs and pour the cheese mixture over the veggies and turkey in the slow cooker.

5. Top the ingredients with shredded cheese and bake them on low until set, preferably overnight. If you like it, use low fat turkey sausage as the crust.

Calories 369.9, Carbs 4.4g, Protein 36.2g, Fat 22.6g

Bacon Bread Sandwich

Prep Time: 5 minutes

Cook Time: 25 minutes

Total Time: 30 minutes

Serves 3

Ingredients

1 tablespoon green onion

2 eggs

6 slices of bacon

Directions

1. First preheat your oven to 450 degrees F.

2. Then cut the bacon slices in half, down the middle using a knife.

3. Intertwine 6 half slices to make a square piece that is 3 by 3 slices.

4. Put both bacon pieces on a baking sheet and cook in a preheated oven for 20 to 30 minutes. Flip once halfway through to cook the other side.

5. In a pan, add in the eggs and fry them sunny side up. Season the eggs with green onion.

6. Once bacon is cooked through, layer the bacon weave with the fried egg and top with the second piece of bacon weave.

Calories 299, Carbs 1.2g, Protein 12.5g, Fat 26.9g

Keto Breakfast Burger

Prep Time: 5 minutes

Cook Time: 20 minutes

Total Time: 25 minutes

Serves 4

Ingredients

8 slices cooked bacon

½-cup sausage, ground

4 eggs

2 tablespoons almond meal

1 pound beef, ground

2 teaspoons basil

1 teaspoon garlic, minced

2-3 sundried tomatoes, sliced

Directions

1. Mix together the turkey or beef meat with one egg, basil, garlic almond meal and the sun dried tomatoes. Form this mixture into 4 burger patties.

2. Then cook bacon if you had it raw, drain it and set aside.

3. Meanwhile, in a skillet, cook the four burger patties for about 5 minutes on each side and set them on plates once cooked through.

4. Then fry the sausage in skillet and top your burgers with the cooked sausage and bacon.

5. Finally fry the 4 eggs one at a time and put them on top of patties. Serve and enjoy.

Calories 804, Carbs 6.1g, Protein 55g, Fat 61g

Keto Sausage Breakfast Sandwich

Prep Time: 5 minutes

Cook Time: 15 minutes

Total Time: 20 minutes

Serves 3

Ingredients

6 frozen sausage patties, heated

3 slices cheddar

1 tablespoon butter

Black pepper, freshly ground

Kosher salt

Pinch red pepper flakes

2 tablespoons heavy cream

6 large eggs

Avocado, sliced

Directions

1. Beat together red pepper flakes, heavy cream and eggs in a small bowl. Season this mixture with pepper and salt.

2. Melt some butter over medium heat in a non-stick skillet. Then pour a third of the eggs into the hot skillet.

3. Add a slice of cheese in the middle of the mixture and allow to melt for a minute. Then fold the sides of the eggs into the center so as to cover the cheese.

4. Once done, remove the sandwich from the pan and repeat the process with the rest of the eggs.

5. Now you can serve the eggs between two sandwiches along with an avocado.

Calories 473, Carb 4g, Protein 22.7g, Fat 40.8g

Breakfast Meat Bagel

Prep Time: 15 minutes

Cook Time: 40 minutes

Total Time: 55 minutes

Serves 4

Ingredients

½ teaspoon pepper

1 teaspoon salt

Paprika

1 teaspoon

2/3 cup tomato sauce

2 large eggs

2 pounds of ground pork

1 tablespoon of butter or bacon fat

1 ½ onions, finely diced

Directions

1. First preheat the oven to 400 degrees F then pick a parchment paper and line a baking dish.

2. Over medium heat, sauté the onion along with cooking fat or bacon grease until translucent. Let the onions cool and then add them to the meat.

3. Mix together all the ingredients in a bowl together with cooked onions. Mix well to blend well with the spices.

4. Now cut the meat into 6 portions and then roll each portion into a ball using your hands. Indent the middle of the ball then flatten slightly to make a bagel.

5. Put the bagel in the dish and repeat the procedure on the other pieces of meat. Bake the bagel until the meat is cooked through, in about 40 minutes.

6. Let the meat bagels cool and then slice them into regular bagel. Fill the bagel with toppings such as onions, lettuce and tomatoes slices.

Calories 767, Carbs 13.7g, Protein 61.3g, Fat 50g

Chicken and Apple Sausage

Prep Time: 15 minutes

Cook Time: 20 minutes

Total Time: 35 minutes

Serves 2-4

Ingredients

3 tablespoons coconut oil

Salt and pepper

2 teaspoons garlic powder

1 tablespoon fresh oregano, finely chopped

3 tablespoons fresh parsley, finely chopped

1 tablespoon fresh thyme leaves, finely chopped

1 apple, peeled and finely diced

1 lb. ground chicken or 2 large chicken breasts

Directions

1. Begin by preheating the oven to 425 degrees F, and then in a skillet, melt 3 tablespoons of coconut oil.

2. Under medium-high heat, cook oregano, parsley, thyme and apples for about 7-8 minutes, or until soft. Cool for 5 minutes.

Keto Diet Breakfast Recipes

3. If using chicken breast, process it and then mix the chicken with the rest of the ingredients in a skillet.

4. Now from the mixture, form 12 and ½-inch-thick patties and position them on a baking tray that is lined with foil.

5. Then bake the patties for about 20 minutes at 170 degrees F and then cool. Keep frozen or refrigerated.

6. In case you need the sausages browned, pan-fry in coconut oil or pan fry raw sausages instead of baking.

7. To serve the sausages, reheat in a microwave or skillet for breakfast.

Calories 345, Carbs 8.9g, Protein 30.9g, Fat 20.4g

Turkey Low Carb Sausage

Prep Time: 5 minutes

Cook Time: 15 minutes

Total Time: 20 minutes

Serves 8

Ingredients

3/4 teaspoon salt

1 pound lean ground turkey

1/2 teaspoon pepper

1/2 teaspoon rubbed sage

1/4 teaspoon ground ginger

Directions

1. First crumble the turkey in a large bowl.

2. Then add the sage, ginger and pepper, and now season with some salt.

3. At this point, mold into 8 two-inch patties, and cook the patties over medium heat in a nonstick skillet that is coated with cooking spray for approximately 4 to 6 minutes.

Calories 85, Carbs 0g, Protein 10g, Fat 5g

Pancakes and Waffles

Fluffy Keto Waffle

Prep Time: 10 minutes

Cook Time: 15 minutes

Total Time: 25 minutes

Serves: 4

Ingredients

Batter:

Almond milk or Half and half as needed

1/2 teaspoon maple extract

1 dash cinnamon

1 1/2 teaspoons baking powder

4 tablespoons coconut flour

1 tablespoon sugar substitute

2 teaspoons vanilla extract, sugar free

4 eggs

4 ounces cream cheese, softened

For pancakes only:

1 tablespoon melted butter

Keto Diet Breakfast Recipes

1/2 teaspoon additional baking powder

1. To make the waffles, mix together eggs, cinnamon, maple extract, sugar substitute, vanilla and cream cheese using a mixer or blender.

2. Then add in melted butter long with coconut flour and baking powder. Blend the mixture until fully incorporated.

3. In case the batter thickened after a few minutes, simply add in a splash of almond milk, half and half and cream to make it thinner. Here, you can choose to either make pancakes or waffles.

4. For pancakes, set the batter on an electric griddle to set to 300 degrees F. Alternatively, heat on a greased pan over medium heat.

5. Now pour the mixture to make circles that are about 4 to 6 inches in diameter.

6. As soon as the surface starts to bubble and the edges begin to harden, flip the pancakes and then cook the other side until golden brown. This should take 2 to 3 minutes.

7. In you choose to make waffles, just add the batter to a preheated iron and cook until golden brown, in about 5 to 7 minutes.

8. Serve the pancakes or waffles with sugar-free syrup or butter.

Calories 200, Carbs 5g, Protein 9g, Fat 15g

Flour-Less Pancakes

Prep Time: 5 minutes

Cook Time: 15 minutes

Total Time: 20 minutes

Serves 2

Ingredients

2 eggs

1 medium ripe banana

Directions

1. In bowl or blender, combine or mash the ingredients together to obtain smooth batter.

2. Over medium heat, pour the batter in a large skillet that is greased with coconut oil.

3. Once the pancakes begin to set and bubble on top, turn and cook the other side. Serve.

Calories 182, Carbs 14.5g, Protein 9.6g, Fat 9.8g

Pancakes with Blueberries

Prep Time: 5 Minutes

Cook Time: 10 minutes

Total Time: 15 minutes

Serves 1

Ingredients

1/4 cup blueberries, fresh

2 tablespoons vanilla whey protein

1/2 ounce curd creamed cottage cheese

1/4 teaspoons baking powder

1/8 cup dry soy flour, whole grain

3/4 large egg

2 tablespoons blanched almond flour

Directions

1. Mix together baking powder, soy flour, protein powder and almond flour.

2. Then stir in the cottage cheese and beaten egg and continue stirring to blend.

3. Over medium heat, heat a large non-stick skillet and use canola oil or butter to lightly grease it.

4. Drop the batter onto the skillet, let's say 1/4 cup per pancake. Flip and then cook the other side as soon as bubbles start to form in the center of each pancake. Cook until firm or for around 2 minutes.

5. You can serve the pancakes with blueberries or add the blueberries to the batter before you cook.

Calories 256.5, Carbs 10.4g, Protein 3.9g, Fat 4.1g

Kitchen Pumpkin Waffles

Prep Time: 5 minutes

Cook Time: 15 minutes

Total Time: 20 minutes

Serves: 5

Ingredients

Maple syrup, for serving

Pinch of fine-grain sea salt

1 teaspoon vanilla extract

1 teaspoon baking powder

1 teaspoon baking soda

2 tablespoons pumpkin pie spice

½ cup coconut flour

¼ cup melted coconut oil,

½ cup almond butter

5 large eggs

½ cup pumpkin puree

2 large bananas, mashed

Directions

Keto Diet Breakfast Recipes

1. Start by preheating the waffle iron.

2. Meanwhile, mix together bananas, coconut oil, almond butter, eggs and pumpkin puree in a food processor or blender and combine to have the mixture blended with all ingredients.

3. When smooth, add in vanilla, baking powder, baking soda, pumpkin pie spice, coconut flour and salt, and then continue to blend until blended.

4. Use some melted coconut oil to lightly brush the waffle iron. Then following package directions of the waffle to get the suggested cup [milliliter] quantity, ladle the batter into your already hot and greased waffle maker.

5. Now spread the batter evenly along the surface. Ensure that you leave about half-an-inch of border, as the batter will spread after closing the lid.

6. Cook the waffle based on the manufacturer's directions, until done. Then set aside onto your plate and keep it warm as you prepare the rest of the waffles.

Calories 394, Carbs 7g, Protein 7.3g, Fats 40.1g

Pecan Hotcakes with Mixed Berries

Prep Time: 15 minutes

Cook Time: 10 minutes

Total Time: 25 minutes

Serves 10

Ingredients

Organic oil or grass-fed butter

1/4 teaspoon pure liquid stevia

1/2 teaspoon baking soda

1/2 teaspoon cinnamon, ground

2 teaspoons pure vanilla extract

4 whole eggs

8 ounces raw pecan pieces

Warmed frozen berries

Directions:

1. Pulse your pecans in a food processor or blender to obtain a fine pecan meal. Pour the pecans into a large mixing bowl and then whisk together with stevia, baking soda, cinnamon, vanilla and eggs.

2. In a pan, warm some butter or oil and then ladle about 2 tablespoons of batter in the pan. Cook the pancake until light

and fluffy on both sides. Your hotcakes should fluff up when cooking.

3. In the microwave or pot, warm the frozen berries and then ladle them onto your hotcakes and serve.

Calories 188, Carbs 3g, Protein 4g, Fat 18g

Blueberries & Cream Crepes

Prep Time: 15 minutes

Cook Time: 10 minutes

Total Time: 25 minutes

Serves 6

Ingredients

1/4 teaspoon baking soda

1/4 teaspoon cinnamon

1/8 teaspoon sea salt

10 drops liquid stevia

2 oz. cream cheese

2 large eggs

For Filling

60 g blueberries

2 tablespoon powdered erythritol

1/2 teaspoon vanilla extract

4 oz. cream cheese

Directions

Keto Diet Breakfast Recipes

1. In a bowl, add egg and cream cheese and then beat the egg using electric hand mixer.

2. Once smooth, add in sea salt, baking soda, cinnamon, stevia and mix well.

3. On medium heat, warm-up a non-stick pan and then add coconut oil or butter. Melt and grease the pan lightly.

4. Pour some batter in the pan, ¼ cup at a time as your swirl it to allow batter spread to the edges.

5. Cook the contents until the edges begin to crisp up, around 3 minutes per crepe. To loosen the crepes, wiggle a spatula around the edges, then under them. Flip and cook the other side.

6. Meanwhile, make the filling by mixing together powdered erythritol, vanilla extract and cream cheese in a bowl.

7. Using an electric mixer, beat the contents until smooth and creamy.

8. After the crepes are done, add the filling to the center of each. Then add blueberries and wrap it up. Serve with extra cinnamon.

Calories 390, Carbs 8g, Protein 13g, Fat 32g

Eggs Benedict Zucchini Pancakes

Prep Time: minutes

Cook Time: minutes

Total Time: minutes

Serves 4

Ingredients

1 tablespoon fresh flat-leaf parsley, chopped

4 zucchini pancakes

4 slices Canadian bacon

4 extra-large eggs, at room temperature

1 tablespoon white vinegar

Directions

1. Preheat your oven to 275 degrees F. Then into a large and shallow saucepan, heat about 3 inches of water over medium heat until bubbles appear around the edges. Now add in the vinegar.

2. Heat 3 inches of water in a separate saucepan to a temperature of 130 degrees F on a candy thermometer. Once hot, remove from heat and cover.

3. Now into a custard cup, break each of the eggs at a time and then slide the eggs from the cup quickly into a barely

simmering vinegar-water. Once all eggs are added, cook for about 2 minutes or until the eggs become too lose.

4. Then lift the barely cooked eggs using a slotted spoon, each egg at a time and then put them into the 130 degrees F boiling water.

5. Cover the mixture and cook for around 15 minutes, while checking the temperatures of the water frequently to ensure its 130 degrees F. In case the temperature drops, add in boiling water to raise the temperature.

6. In a large non-stick frying pan, put Canadian bacon over medium heat and fry it, as you turn it regularly. Cook for 4 minutes to have it just turns light brown around the edges.

7. Then remove the meat from heat and now put onto a baking sheet that has been placed in a preheated oven to maintain warmth, in case pancakes and eggs aren't done yet.

8. At the center of each plate, put a warm pancake and then top with a slice of Canadian bacon. Lift the poached eggs using the slotted spoon from the water, one at a time; and use a kitchen towel to pat and dry the excess water.

9. Now put an egg on top of the bacon. In case the eggs edges are rugged, use a small knife or kitchen knife to carefully trim.

10. Finally sprinkle about 3 tablespoons of hollandaise sauce on top of each egg, and then sprinkle a little amount of chopped parsley. Serve the breakfast immediately.

Keto Diet Breakfast Recipes

Calories 200, Carbs 6.3g, Protein 14.3g, Fat 8.4g

Conclusion

As you can see, breakfast doesn't have to be same old unappetizing foods as far as Ketogenic diet is concerned. Now go out and buy the required ingredients so that you can try out these delicious recipes in whichever order you prefer! All you need to do is to try as many recipes as you can so that you find which ones you find most delicious then you can come up with your own go-to recipes, which you can prepare as often as possible.

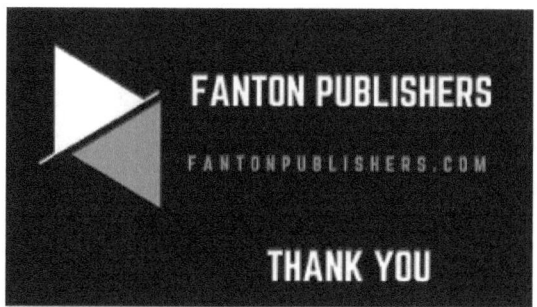

Do You Like My Book & Approach To Publishing?

If you like my writing and style and would love the ease of learning literally everything you can get your hands on from Fantonpublishers.com, I'd really need you to do me either of the following favors.

1: First, I'd Love It If You Leave a Review of This Book on Amazon.

2: Check Out My Other Keto Diet Books

KETOGENIC DIET: Keto Diet Made Easy: Beginners Guide on How to Burn Fat Fast With the Keto Diet (Including 100+ Recipes That You Can Prepare Within 20 Minutes)- New Edition

KETOGENIC DIET: Ketogenic Diet Recipes That You Can Prepare Using 7 Ingredients and Less in Less Than 30 Minutes

Ketogenic Diet: With A Sustainable Twist: Lose Weight Rapidly With Ketogenic Diet Recipes You Can Make Within 25 Minutes

Ketogenic Diet: Keto Diet Breakfast Recipes

Fat Bombs: Keto Fat Bombs: 50+ Savory and Sweet Ketogenic Diet Fat Bombs That You MUST Prepare Before Any Other!

Snacks: Keto Diet Snacks: 50+ Savory and Sweet Ketogenic Diet Snacks That You MUST Prepare Before Any Other!

Desserts: Keto Diet Desserts: 50+ Savory and Sweet Ketogenic Diet Desserts That You MUST Prepare Before Any Other!

Ketogenic Diet: Ketogenic Diet Lunch and Dinner Recipes

Ketogenic Diet: Keto Diet Cookbook For Vegetarians

Ketogenic Diet: Ketogenic Slow Cooker Cookbook: Keto Slow Cooker Recipes That You Can Prepare Using 7 Ingredients Or Less

Note: This list may not represent all my Keto diet books. You can check the full list by visiting my Author Central: amazon.com/author/fantonpublishers or my website http://www.fantonpublishers.com

Get updates when we publish any book on the Ketogenic diet: http://bit.ly/2fantonpubketo

Closely related to the keto diet is intermittent fasting. I also publish books on Intermittent Fasting.

One of the books is shown below:

Intermittent Fasting: A Complete Beginners Guide to Intermittent Fasting For Weight Loss, Increased Energy, and A Healthy Life

Get updates when we publish any book on intermittent fasting: http://bit.ly/2fantonbooksIF

To get a list of all my other books, please fantonwriters.com, my author central or let me send you the list by requesting them below: http://bit.ly/2fantonpubnewbooks

3: Let's Get In Touch

Antony

Website: http://www.fantonpublishers.com/

Email: Support@fantonpublishers.com

Twitter: https://twitter.com/FantonPublisher

Facebook Page: https://www.facebook.com/Fantonpublisher/

My Ketogenic Diet Books Page: https://www.facebook.com/pg/Fast-Keto-Meals-336338180266944

Private Facebook Group For Readers: https://www.facebook.com/groups/FantonPublishers/

Pinterest: https://www.pinterest.com/fantonpublisher/

4: Grab Some Freebies On Your Way Out; Giving Is Receiving, Right?

I gave you 2 freebies at the start of the book, one on general life transformation and one about the Ketogenic diet. Grab them here if you didn't grab them earlier.

Ketogenic Diet Freebie: http://bit.ly/2fantonpubketo

5 Pillar Life Transformation Checklist: http://bit.ly/2fantonfreebie

5: Suggest Topics That You'd Love Me To Cover To Increase Your Knowledge Bank.

I am looking forward to seeing your suggestions and insights; you could even suggest improvements to this book. Simply send me a message on Support@fantonpublishers.com.

PSS: Let Me Also Help You Save Some Money!

If you are a heavy reader, have you considered subscribing to Kindle Unlimited? You can read this and millions of other books for just $9.99 a month)! You can check it out by searching for Kindle Unlimited on Amazon!